CHAIR YOGA SLIM DOWN

EFFECTIVE PRACTICES FOR WEIGHT LOSS

By

Asuncion M. McGinnis

TABLE OF CONTENTS

"Chair Yoga Slim Down: Effective Practices for Weight Loss." We shall begin on a journey to uncover the transformational potential of chair yoga in the process of attaining your weight reduction objectives during the course of this article. Chair yoga is a mild yet effective method of exercise that can be modified to any fitness level and physical condition. It is applicable to individuals who are new to yoga as well as those who have been practicing yoga for a long time.

Let's take a minute to familiarize ourselves with the concept of chair yoga and the ways in which it may be beneficial to you before we get into the details of chair yoga for weight reduction. One type of yoga is called chair yoga, and it is performed by sitting on a chair or utilizing a chair as a support while performing the poses. Meditation methods, mild stretches, and breathing exercises are all incorporated into this practice in order to enhance both physical and mental well-being.

It is one of the most significant advantages of chair yoga because it is easily accessible. Chair yoga is a kind of yoga that may be done by anyone of any age or ability, including those who have mobility challenges, injuries, or chronic diseases. This is in contrast to conventional yoga, which typically requires participants to get down on the floor. By completing yoga postures while seated or utilizing a chair for support, you may experience the benefits of yoga without placing strain on your joints or risking injury.

But what makes chair yoga particularly good for weight loss? The solution lies in its ability to target crucial parts of the body that are typically missed in regular training programs. Through a mix of moderate stretches, strength-building postures, and attentive breathing, chair yoga can help you build lean muscle mass, improve flexibility, and boost circulation – all of which are necessary for burning calories and reducing extra weight.

In addition to its physical benefits, chair yoga also offers several mental and emotional benefits that can help your weight reduction journey. By practicing mindfulness and meditation techniques, you may learn to create a stronger sense of self-awareness and self-compassion, which are vital for making good lifestyle choices and maintaining long-term weight reduction success.

Throughout this book, we will study the science behind weight reduction and how chair yoga may contribute to your overall fitness and well-being. We will present a complete introduction to chair yoga postures particularly aimed for weight reduction, along with sample routines tailored to help you accomplish your objectives. Whether you're wanting to thin down, tone up, or simply improve your overall health, chair yoga offers a safe, effective, and pleasurable approach to attain your fitness objectives.

But maybe most significantly, this book is about enabling you to take responsibility of your health and well-being. It's about realizing that you have the capacity to create great changes in your life, no matter where you're starting from or what challenges you may face. By adding chair yoga into your daily routine, you may create a better feeling of vigor, resilience, and joy — not only in your body, but in your mind and soul as well.

So, are you ready to begin on this trip with us? Are you ready to explore the revolutionary potential of chair yoga for weight loss? If yes, then let's begin. Let's take the first step towards a healthier, happier, and more vibrant self. Together, we can attain our goals and release our entire potential. Let's make every breath count, every stretch count, and every moment count. Let's make chair yoga slim down a reality.

This introduction sets the tone for the rest of the book by offering an outline of what readers may expect to learn and achieve via practicing chair yoga for weight reduction. It demonstrates the value of chair yoga as an accessible and effective exercise technique and urges readers to engage in the path towards greater health and well-being.

CHAPTER 1.

UNDERSTANDING CHAIR YOGA

Chair yoga is a moderate type of yoga that is conducted while seated on a chair or utilizing a chair for support. It offers a simplified approach to conventional yoga positions, making it accessible to persons of different ages, fitness levels, and physical problems. In this part, we'll discuss what chair yoga is, its history and origins, the advantages it gives, and how it varies from traditional yoga.

WHAT IS CHAIR YOGA?

Chair yoga is a kind of yoga that modifies classic yoga poses and practices to be practiced while seated or utilizing a chair for support. Meditation methods, mild stretches, and breathing exercises are all incorporated into this practice in order to enhance both physical and mental well-being. Chair yoga is especially popular among elders, persons with mobility difficulties, injuries, or chronic diseases, and others who may find regular yoga tough.

In chair yoga, the chair provides as a sturdy basis for executing various yoga postures, allowing practitioners to safely and comfortably explore movement and breath. The practice focuses on increasing flexibility, improving posture, boosting strength, and enhancing relaxation and awareness. Chair yoga may be done in a number of venues, including at home, in the workplace, or in community centers, making it accessible to individuals from all walks of life.

HISTORY AND ORIGINS OF CHAIR YOGA

While the specific roots of chair yoga are obscure, the practice may be traced back to the principles of classical yoga. In ancient times, yoga was predominantly done in sat or reclining positions, with the purpose of promoting inner tranquility, self-awareness, and spiritual enlightenment. Over time, yoga expanded to include more dynamic and physically demanding poses, yet the practice of sitting yoga survived.

In the contemporary period, the notion of chair yoga gained popularity as a technique to make yoga more accessible to a larger audience. The credit for popularizing chair yoga is frequently credited to Lakshmi Voelker-Binder, a yoga instructor who established a chair yoga curriculum in the 1980s to accommodate her pupils with mobility limitations. Since then, chair yoga has continued to grow in popularity, with many instructors and practitioners throughout the world embracing its gentle and inclusive approach to yoga.

BENEFITS OF CHAIR YOGA

Chair yoga offers a wide range of physical, mental, and emotional advantages for practitioners of all ages and abilities. Some of the primary benefits of chair yoga include:

1. **Improved flexibility**: Chair yoga poses gently stretch and mobilize the muscles and joints, helping to enhance range of motion and flexibility.

2. **Enhanced strength**: Many chair yoga poses involve resistance and weight-bearing aspects, which can assist to increase strength and stability, particularly in the core, arms, and legs.

3. **Better posture:** Chair yoga fosters optimal alignment and spinal awareness, leading to improved posture and reduced risk of back discomfort and postural imbalances.

4. **Stress relief**: Chair yoga integrates breathwork and relaxation techniques to encourage stress reduction and mental relaxation, helping to calm the mind and soothe the nervous system.

5. **Increased circulation**: The gentle motions and stretches of chair yoga can assist to enhance blood flow and circulation throughout the body, boosting overall health and vitality.

6. **Mindfulness and focus:** Chair yoga emphasizes present-moment mindfulness and focused breathing, generating a sense

of inner serenity, concentration, and mental clarity.

7. **Accessibility**: One of the main benefits of chair yoga is its accessibility. The practice may be adapted to accommodate persons with mobility difficulties, injuries, or chronic diseases, making it suited for people of all ages and fitness levels.

HOW CHAIR YOGA DIFFERS FROM TRADITIONAL YOGA

While chair yoga shares many parallels with conventional yoga, there are several crucial characteristics that set it apart.

Here are a few ways in which chair yoga varies from conventional yoga:

1. **Seated postures**: In chair yoga, most poses are performed while seated on a chair or utilizing a chair for support. Traditional yoga, on the other hand, often incorporates a combination of sitting, standing, and reclining positions.

2. **changed positions**: Chair yoga poses are typically changed to be more accessible and pleasant for those with mobility concerns or physical limitations. Traditional yoga positions may be more dynamic and physically demanding,

requiring greater flexibility, strength, and balance.

3. **Use of props**: In chair yoga, props such as chairs, blocks, and straps are utilized to offer support and aid in executing postures. Traditional yoga may also include props, although they are often less popular and may not be as fundamental to the practice.

4. **Focus on breathwork and mindfulness**: Chair yoga offers a significant focus on breath awareness and mindfulness, with an emphasis on calm, deliberate breathing and present-moment

awareness. While conventional yoga also contains breathwork and mindfulness, chair yoga frequently simplifies and accentuates these parts of the practice to make them more accessible to beginners and persons with restricted mobility.

CHAPTER 2

THE SCIENCE OF WEIGHT LOSS

In this section, we will dig into the science of weight reduction, investigating the principles and mechanisms that regulate the body's capacity to shed weight. Understanding the science of weight reduction is vital for designing successful plans and procedures to reach and maintain a healthy weight.

PRINCIPLES OF WEIGHT LOSS

At its foundation, weight reduction is a simple equation: calories in vs calories out. When you consume less calories than your body requires to maintain its present weight, you generate a calorie deficit, which leads to weight loss. Conversely, when you consume more calories than your body requires, you develop a calorie surplus, which contributes to weight gain.

However, the human body is a complicated system, and weight reduction is impacted by a multitude of variables beyond basic calorie tracking. Hormones, metabolism, heredity, and environmental variables all play a part in determining how effectively your body burns calories and stores fat.

ENERGY BALANCE AND METABOLISM

Energy balance refers to the balance between the calories you ingest via food and beverages and the calories you expend through physical activity and fundamental metabolic operations. When you create a calorie deficit by ingesting fewer calories than you spend, your body draws into its energy stores (stored fat) to make up the difference, leading to weight loss.

Metabolism, or the pace at which your body consumes calories to support essential physiological activities such as breathing, digestion, and circulation, also plays a vital part in weight reduction. Metabolism can vary greatly from person to person and is impacted by factors such as age, sex, muscle mass, and thyroid function. While some people have a naturally high metabolism that allows them to burn calories more effectively, others may have a slower metabolism that makes weight reduction more tough.

TYPES OF FAT

Not all fat is created equal. The body stores fat in two primary forms: subcutaneous fat, which is found just beneath the skin, and visceral fat, which is deposited deep inside the abdominal cavity and surrounds critical organs such as the liver, pancreas, and intestines.

Visceral fat, commonly known as belly fat, is particularly worrying from a health viewpoint, since it has been related to an increased risk of chronic illnesses such as heart disease, type 2 diabetes, and certain forms of cancer. Losing extra visceral fat through weight reduction can improve health outcomes and lessen the likelihood of acquiring certain illnesses.

FACTORS AFFECTING WEIGHT LOSS

While generating a calorie deficit is the core premise of weight reduction, various factors might impact how successfully you lose weight and retain your results:

1. **Diet composition:** The sorts of meals you eat might effect your weight reduction results. A diet rich in whole, nutrient-dense foods such as fruits, vegetables, lean meats, and whole grains is related with higher weight reduction and better overall

health outcomes compared to a diet high in processed foods, refined sugars, and harmful fats.

2. **Physical activity**: Regular exercise is necessary for attaining and maintaining weight loss. Physical exercise not only burns calories but also helps to grow lean muscle mass, which raises metabolism and improves overall body composition. Incorporating both aerobic exercise and strength training into your fitness program helps enhance weight reduction outcomes.

3. **Sleep quality**: Poor sleep quality and poor sleep duration have been related to

weight growth and obesity. Sleep deprivation can affect hormones that control appetite and metabolism, leading to increased hunger and desires for unhealthy foods. Prioritizing quality sleep and aiming for 7-9 hours of sleep every night can improve weight reduction attempts.

4. **Stress management**: Chronic stress can cause the production of cortisol, a hormone that increases fat accumulation, especially around the abdomen area. Learning effective stress management practices such as mindfulness, meditation, yoga, and deep breathing exercises can

help lower stress levels and assist weight reduction.

5. **Genetics**: Genetics have a key part in defining an individual's tendency to weight gain and obesity. Some people may have genetic traits that make it more difficult for them to lose weight or sustain weight reduction, while others may have genetic advantages that favor a leaner body composition. However, genetics are not destiny, and lifestyle factors such as food, exercise, and stress management can still exert a major effect on weight reduction outcomes.

THE ROLE OF CHAIR YOGA IN WEIGHT LOSS

Now that we've covered the science underlying weight reduction, let's evaluate how chair yoga may contribute to your weight loss journey. While chair yoga may not burn as many calories as high-intensity cardiovascular exercise or strength training, it offers a range of physical, mental, and emotional advantages that can promote weight reduction in diverse ways.

1. **Increased calorie expenditure**: While chair yoga may not be as calorie-intensive as other kinds of exercise, it nevertheless burns calories and contributes to total

energy expenditure. The moderate motions and stretches of chair yoga work various muscle groups and boost heart rate, leading to higher calorie burn over time.

2. **Improved metabolism:** Regular physical exercise, such as chair yoga, can enhance metabolism and increase the body's capacity to burn calories during rest. By developing lean muscular strength and boosting cardiovascular health, chair yoga helps to enhance metabolic function and promote weight loss attempts.

3. **Stress reduction**: Stress is a major cause for emotional eating and bad food

choices, which can derail weight loss attempts. Chair yoga combines relaxation methods such as deep breathing, mindfulness, and meditation, which assist to lower stress levels and create a sense of serenity and well-being.

4. **Mindful eating**: Chair yoga cultivates present-moment focus and mindfulness, which may extend to other areas of life, including eating habits. By practicing mindfulness during chair yoga sessions, you can build a deeper awareness of hunger and satiety cues, making it easier to make intentional, wholesome meal choices that assist weight reduction.

5. **Improved body awareness**: Chair yoga fosters perfect alignment, posture, and body awareness, helping you to build a stronger feeling of connection to your body and its needs. By listening into your body's signals and practicing self-care and self-compassion, you may build a healthy connection with food, exercise, and body image that promotes sustained weight reduction.

chair yoga offers a comprehensive approach to weight management that tackles not only the physical components of fitness but also the mental and emotional variables that impact eating choices and body composition. By including chair yoga into your daily routine, you may harness its transforming potential to reach your weight reduction goals and create a better, happier connection with your body.

This part gives a deep investigation of the science behind weight reduction, covering subjects such as energy balance, metabolism, forms of fat, and variables impacting weight loss success. It also stresses the significance of chair yoga in helping weight reduction attempts and gives practical insights into how chair yoga may contribute to a healthy lifestyle.

CHAPTER 3

GETTING STARTED WITH CHAIR YOGA

In this part, we'll discuss how to get started with chair yoga, including setting up your area, learning basic principles, and practicing core postures. Whether you're new to yoga or seeking for a moderate method to include movement into your daily routine, chair yoga offers an accessible and pleasurable choice for people of all ages and fitness levels.

SETTING UP YOUR SPACE

Before you begin practicing chair yoga, it's crucial to create a comfortable and appealing setting where you can focus and relax. Here are some recommendations for setting up your chair yoga space:

1. Choose a calm and clutter-free environment where you won't be bothered throughout your practice.

2. Find a robust chair with a flat seat and backrest that gives support and stability. Avoid chairs with wheels or arms that may hinder mobility.

3. Place your chair on a non-slip surface such as a yoga mat or carpet to prevent it from slipping or tipping over during postures.

4. Gather any props or accessories you may need, such as yoga blocks, blankets, or straps, and place them within easy reach.

5. Adjust the height of your chair as needed to ensure that your feet are flat on the floor and your knees are aligned with your hips while seated.

Once you've set up your environment, take a minute to focus yourself and ready for your practice. Sit comfortably in your chair with your feet flat on the floor and your spine tall and straight. Close your eyes and take a few deep breaths, inhaling with your nose and expelling through your mouth, to calm your thoughts and connect with your breath.

UNDERSTANDING BASIC PRINCIPLES

Before we dig into particular postures and sequences, let's take a time to review the basic concepts of chair yoga:

1. **Listen to your body**: In chair yoga, it's crucial to listen to your body and acknowledge its limitations. If a position is uncomfortable or causes pain, back off and adapt as required. Never force yourself into a stance or push beyond your edge.

2. **Breathe mindfully:** Breath is a vital aspect of yoga, helping to relax the mind, manage energy, and assist movement. Focus on breathing deeply and evenly throughout your practice, inhaling and expelling through the nose with mindfulness and intention.

3. **Practice with intention**: Every posture in chair yoga gives a chance to enhance presence, awareness, and mindfulness. Approach your practice with curiosity and openness, allowing each breath and movement to bring you deeper into the present now.

4. **Modify and adapt**: Chair yoga postures may be tweaked and altered to fit your specific requirements and skills. Don't be hesitant to utilize props, modify your placement, or omit poses completely if they don't feel right for your body.

5. **Stay present**: Chair yoga is not just about physical movement; it's also about fostering mental and emotional awareness. Stay present with your thoughts and feelings while you practice, detecting any areas of tension or resistance and gently releasing them with each breath.

By keeping these ideas in mind as you practice chair yoga, you may create a safe, engaging, and productive experience that promotes your overall health and well-being.

PRACTICING FOUNDATIONAL POSES

For the sake of getting you started with chair yoga, let's take a look at some core postures now that you are familiar with the fundamentals of the practice. These postures are designed to stretch and move the body in a gentle manner, to improve circulation, to induce relaxation, and to alleviate tension.

1. Sit up straight in your chair and assume the seated mountain pose, also known as Tadasana. Place your feet firmly on the ground and keep your spine straight. Lie down on your knees or thighs with your

palms facing down. Rest your hands there. You should close your eyes and take a few deep breaths, focusing on grounding yourself via your sit bones and working your way up to the crown of your head.

2. Passimottanasana, also known as the Seated Forward Fold, requires you to sit up straight in your chair with your feet hip-width apart. When you inhale, your spine will be extended, and when you exhale, you will tilt forward from your hips, bringing your chest closer to your thighs. Your head and neck should be relaxed, and you should allow your hands to rest on your shins or the floor nearby.

Hold for a few breaths, then inhale to rise back up.

3. Seated Twist (Ardha Matsyendrasana): Sit up straight in your chair with your feet planted firmly on the ground and your spine in a straight straight line. Make sure that your left hand is resting on the outside of your right leg and that your right hand is resting on the back of the chair. Inhale to stretch your spine, and then exhale to rotate to the right at the same time. Hold for a few breaths, then inhale to return to center and repeat on the opposing side.

4. Seated Cat-Cow Stretch: Sit tall in your chair with your feet flat on the floor and your hands resting on your thighs. Inhale to arch your back and raise your chest towards the ceiling (Cow), then exhale to circle your spine and tuck your chin into your chest (Cat). Continue to move between these two postures with your breath, moving easily and mindfully.

5. Seated Ankle Rolls: Sit tall in your chair with your feet flat on the floor. Lift your right foot off the floor and begin to circle your ankle in one direction, moving softly and with control. After a few

rotations, shift directions and continue to circle your ankle. Repeat on the left side.

This section includes a full introduction to beginning began with chair yoga, including guidelines for setting up your location, learning essential ideas, and practicing core poses. By following these instructions, you may begin to explore the transforming potential of chair yoga and experience its myriad benefits for your body, mind, and spirit.

CHAPTER 4

CHAIR YOGA POSES FOR WEIGHT LOSS

In this segment, we'll cover a number of chair yoga poses particularly designed to encourage weight loss. These postures focus on improving strength, increasing flexibility, enhancing circulation, and decreasing stress—all of which can contribute to a healthier body composition and a more balanced metabolism. Whether you're new to chair yoga or a seasoned practitioner, these poses offer accessible and effective tools for enhancing your weight loss journey.

1.   Seated   Forward   Fold (Paschimottanasana)

- • - Begin by sitting tall in your chair with your feet hip-width apart and your spine straight.

- • - Inhale to stretch your spine, then exhale to lean forward from your hips, bringing your chest towards your thighs.

- • - Allow your hands to rest on your shins or the floor, and relax your head and neck.

- • - Hold the pose for 5-10 breaths, focussing on increasing the stretch with each exhale.

- • - To come out of the posture, inhale to slowly raise back up to a sitting position.

BENEFITS:

- • - Stretches the hamstrings, lower back, and spine.

- ● - Stimulates digestion and metabolism.

- ● - Calms the mind and reduces tension.

2. Seated Twist (Ardha Matsyendrasan)

- ● - Begin by sitting tall in your chair with your feet flat on the floor and your spine straight.

- ● - Inhale to stretch your spine, then exhale to twist to the right, placing your left hand on the outside of your

right thigh and your right hand on
the back of the chair.

- - Gently press into the chair with
  your right palm to deepen the twist,
  and move your gaze over your right
  shoulder.

- - Hold the position for 5-10 breaths,
  feeling the twist from your belly
  button up to your shoulders.

- - To come out of the posture, inhale
  to softly return to center, then repeat
  on the opposing side.

BENEFITS:

- - Increases spinal mobility and flexibility.

- - Stimulates the digestive organs and aids in detoxifying.

- - Energizes the body and promotes circulation.

3. Chair Warrior I (Virabhadrasana I)

- - Begin by sitting tall in your chair with your feet hip-width apart and your spine straight.

- ● - Step your right foot back behind you, keeping your toes pointed forward and your heel lifted.

- ● - Inhale to stretch your arms upwards, bringing your palms together.

- ● - Exhale to bend your left knee, lowering your hips down and forward into a lunge position.

- ● - Keep your chest lifted and your gaze ahead, engaging your core and pressing firmly into your feet.

- • - Hold the pose for 5-10 breaths, getting a stretch through your hips and thighs.

- • - To come out of the posture, inhale to straighten your left leg and return to a sitting position, then repeat on the opposite side.

BENEFITS:

- • - Strengthens the legs, glutes, and core muscles.

- • - Improves balance and stability.

- • - Builds mental focus and concentration.

4. Chair Warrior II (Virabhadrasana II)

- • - Begin by sitting tall in your chair with your feet hip-width apart and your spine straight.

- • - Step your right foot back behind you, keeping your toes pointing forward and your heel raised.

- • - Inhale to stretch your arms out to the sides, parallel to the floor, with your palms facing down.

- - Exhale to bend your left knee, bringing it directly over your ankle, and move your eyes over your left hand.

- - Keep your shoulders relaxed and your chest open, engaging your core and pushing firmly into your feet.

- - Hold the stance for 5-10 breaths, experiencing a stretch across your inner thighs and groin.

- - To come out of the posture, inhale to straighten your left leg and return to a sitting position, then repeat on the opposite side.

BENEFITS:

- Opens the hips and chest.

- Improves circulation and respiration.

- Enhances attention and concentration.

5. Chair Cat-Cow Stretch

- - Begin by sitting tall in your chair with your feet flat on the floor and your hands resting on your thighs.

- - Inhale to arch your back and elevate your chest towards the ceiling (Cow), pulling your shoulder blades together.

- - Exhale to circle your spine and tuck your chin into your chest (Cat), squeezing your hands into your thighs and rounding your upper back.

- - Continue to move between these two postures with your breath, flowing naturally and attentively.

- - Repeat for 5-10 rounds, focusing on matching your movement with your breath.

- - To come out of the posture, inhale to return to a neutral spine and relax for a few breaths before going on to the next pose.

BENEFITS:

- - Improves spinal flexibility and mobility.
- - Strengthens the core and abdominal muscles.
- - Relieves tension and stress in the back and neck.

6. Chair Boat Pose (Navasana)

- • - Begin by sitting tall in your chair with your feet flat on the floor and your spine straight.

- • - Lean back slightly and elevate your feet off the floor, bringing your shins parallel to the ground.

- • - Engage your core and stretch your arms forward, reaching them alongside your legs.

- ● - Keep your chest raised and your shoulders relaxed, striking a balance between effort and ease.

- ● - Hold the stance for 5-10 breaths, feeling your abdominal muscles engage and your breath deepen.

- ● - To come out of the posture, exhale to lower your feet back to the floor and return to a sitting position.

BENEFITS:

- ● - Strengthens the core muscles, especially the abdominals and hip flexors.

- - Improves balance and stability.

- - Stimulates digestion and metabolism.

7. Chair Tree Pose (Vrksasana)

- - Begin by sitting tall in your chair with your feet flat on the floor and your spine straight.

- - Shift your weight into your left foot and lift your right foot off the floor, putting the sole of your right foot against the inner of your left thigh or calf.

- - Press your foot firmly into your leg and your leg back into your foot, establishing a secure and balanced position.

- - Bring your hands together at your heart center, or stretch them overhead for an extra challenge.

- - Hold the posture for 5-10 breaths, feeling anchored and grounded through your standing leg.

- - To come out of the posture, exhale to lower your right foot back to the floor and return to a sitting position, then repeat on the other side.

BENEFITS:

- - Improves balance and focus.
- - Strengthens the muscles of the legs and ankles.
- - Increases flexibility in the hips and groin.

Incorporating chair yoga postures into your daily routine can be an excellent method to assist your weight reduction goals and increase your general well-being. By practicing these positions frequently, you may build strength, flexibility, and awareness, while lowering tension and increasing relaxation. Whether you're wanting to augment your present workout regimen or explore a mild form of movement, chair yoga provides accessible and entertaining solutions for people of all ages and fitness levels.

This section gives a complete reference to chair yoga positions for weight reduction, giving step-by-step directions, benefits, and adjustments for each pose. By adding these postures into your daily routine, you may harness the transforming power of yoga to assist your weight loss journey and create a better, happier relationship with your body and mind.

CHAPTER 5

CHAIR YOGA ROUTINES FOR WEIGHT LOSS

In this part, we'll examine a range of chair yoga exercises specifically intended to promote weight reduction. These routines blend moderate exercises, deep breathing, and mindfulness techniques to help you gain strength, enhance flexibility, and improve circulation—all of which are vital components of a successful weight reduction program. Whether you're new to chair yoga or a seasoned practitioner, these practices offer accessible and efficient tools for optimizing your weight reduction journey.

Routine 1: Gentle Stretch and Mobilize
This program focuses on mild stretches and mobilizing motions to assist develop flexibility, improve circulation, and release tension in the body.

1. Seated Cat-Cow Stretch:
- • - Begin by sitting tall in your chair with your feet flat on the floor and your hands resting on your thighs.

- - Inhale to arch your back and elevate your chest towards the ceiling (Cow), pulling your shoulder blades together.

- - Exhale to circle your spine and tuck your chin into your chest (Cat), squeezing your hands into your thighs and rounding your upper back.

- - Continue to move between these two postures with your breath, flowing naturally and attentively.

- - Repeat for 5-10 rounds, focusing on matching your movement with your breath.

2. Seated Side Stretch:

- - Sit tall in your chair with your feet flat on the floor and your spine straight.

- - Inhale to stretch your arms overhead, interlocking your fingers and pressing your palms towards the ceiling.

* - Exhale to lean slightly to the right, extending through the left side of your body.

* - Hold the stretch for 3-5 breaths, feeling a growing sensation of extending through the left side.

* - Inhale to return to center, then exhale to repeat on the other side.

3. Seated Spinal Twist:
* - Sit tall in your chair with your feet flat on the floor and your spine straight.

- - Inhale to extend your spine, then exhale to twist to the right, placing your left hand on the outside of your right leg and your right hand on the back of the chair.

- - Gently press into the chair with your right hand to deepen the twist, and turn your eyes over your right shoulder.

- - Hold the position for 3-5 breaths, experiencing a gently wringing out sensation across the spine.

- - Inhale to return to center, then exhale to repeat on the other side.

4. Seated Forward Fold:

- - Sit tall in your chair with your feet hip-width apart and your spine straight.

- - Inhale to extend your spine, then exhale to tilt forward from your hips, bringing your chest towards your thighs.

- - Allow your hands to rest on your shins or the floor, and relax your head and neck.

- ● - Hold the posture for 3-5 breaths, experiencing a stretch through the hamstrings and lower back.

- ● - Inhale to slowly climb back up to a sitting position.

5. Seated Ankle Rolls:

- ● - Sit tall on your chair with your feet flat on the floor.

- ● - Lift your right foot off the floor and begin to circle your ankle in one direction, moving carefully and with control.

- - After a few circles, swap directions and continue to circle your ankle.

- - Repeat on the left side, circling the ankle in both directions.

Routine 2: Energize and Activate

This program emphasizes on stimulating and engaging the body, improving metabolism, and promoting circulation.

1. Seated Mountain Pose:
   - - Begin by sitting tall in your chair with your feet flat on the floor and your spine straight.

- - Inhale to stretch your arms above, bringing your palms together.

- - Exhale to push your palms together and focus your core, elevating your chest towards the ceiling.

- - Hold the posture for 3-5 breaths, experiencing a sensation of strength and stability through the spine.

- - Inhale to lower your arms back down to your sides.

2. Chair Warrior II:

- • - Sit tall in your chair with your feet hip-width apart and your spine straight.

- • - Step your right foot back behind you, keeping your toes pointing forward and your heel raised.

- • - Inhale to stretch your arms out to the sides, parallel to the floor, with your palms facing down.

- • - Exhale to bend your left knee, bringing it directly over your ankle, and move your eyes over your left hand.

- • - Hold the posture for 3-5 breaths, experiencing a sensation of strength and stability through the legs and core.

- • - Inhale to straighten your left leg and return to a sitting position, then repeat on the opposite side.

3. Seated Chair Pose:
- • - Begin by sitting tall in your chair with your feet flat on the floor and your spine straight.

- - Inhale to stretch your arms above, bringing your palms together.

- - Exhale to bend your knees and sink your hips down and back, as if sitting into an imagined chair.

- - Hold the posture for 3-5 breaths, experiencing a sensation of power and engagement through the legs and core.

- - Inhale to raise back up to a sitting position.

4. Seated Boat Pose

- - Sit tall in your chair with your feet flat on the floor and your spine straight.

- - Lean back slightly and elevate your feet off the floor, bringing your shins parallel to the ground.

- - Engage your core and stretch your arms forward, reaching them alongside your legs.

- - Hold the posture for 3-5 breaths, feeling a sensation of activation and engagement through the core and legs.

- - Exhale to lower your feet back to the floor and return to a sitting position.

5. Seated Sun Salutation:
- - Begin by sitting tall in your chair with your feet flat on the floor and your hands resting on your thighs.

- - Inhale to stretch your arms above, bringing your palms together.
- - Exhale to tilt forward from your hips, bringing your chest towards

your thighs and your hands towards the floor.

- Inhale to stretch your spine and pull your chest forward, entering into a sitting backbend.

- • - Exhale to circle your spine and lower your chin into your chest, going into a sitting forward fold.

- • - Continue to go through this cycle with your breath, flowing naturally and attentively.

Routine 3: Relax and Restore

This program focuses on relaxation and restoration, helping to reduce stress, quiet the mind, and enhance general well-being.

1. Seated Forward Fold with Shoulder Opener:

- • - Begin by sitting tall in your chair with your feet hip-width apart and your spine straight.

- • - Inhale to stretch your arms above, bringing your palms together.

- • - Exhale to tilt forward from your hips, bringing your chest towards

your thighs and your hands towards
the floor.

- - Allow your head to hang heavy and
your shoulders to relax.

- - Hold the position for 3-5 breaths,
experiencing a deep stretch through
the spine and shoulders.

- - Inhale to slowly climb back up to a
sitting position.

2. Seated Cat-Cow Stretch with Neck Release:

- • - Begin by sitting tall in your chair with your feet flat on the floor and your hands resting on your thighs.

- • - Inhale to arch your back and elevate your chest towards the ceiling (Cow), pulling your shoulder blades together.

- • - Exhale to circle your spine and tuck your chin into your chest (Cat), squeezing your hands into your thighs and rounding your upper back.

- - Continue to move between these two postures with your breath, flowing naturally and attentively.

- - After a few rounds, add a mild neck release by dropping your right ear towards your right shoulder and holding for a few breaths, then repeating on the left side.

3. Seated Twist with Side Body Stretch:
- - Begin by sitting tall in your chair with your feet flat on the floor and your spine straight.

- - Inhale to extend your spine, then exhale to twist to the right, placing your left hand on the outside of your right leg and your right hand on the back of the chair.

- - Gently press into the chair with your right hand to deepen the twist, and turn your eyes over your right shoulder.

- - Hold the position for 3-5 breaths, experiencing a gently wringing out sensation across the spine.

- ● - Inhale to return to center, then exhale to reach your left arm up and over your head, stretching through the left side of your body.

- ● - Hold for 3-5 breaths, feeling a growing sensation of extending across the side body.

- ● - Inhale to return to center, then exhale to repeat on the other side.

4. Seated Pigeon Pose with Forward Fold:
- ● - Begin by sitting tall in your chair with your feet flat on the floor and your spine straight.

- - Inhale to cross your right ankle over your left knee, flexing your right foot.

- - Exhale to tilt forward from your hips, bringing your chest towards your thighs and your hands towards the floor.

- - Allow your head to hang heavy and your shoulders to relax.

- - Hold the position for 3-5 breaths, experiencing a deep stretch across the outer hip and glute.

- - Inhale to gently raise back up to a sitting position, then repeat on the opposite side.

5. Seated Relaxation Pose:

- - Sit tall in your chair with your feet flat on the floor and your hands resting on your thighs.

- - Close your eyes and take a few deep breaths, inhaling through your nose and expelling through your mouth.

- - Allow your body to relax completely, releasing any tension or tightness with each breath.

- - Stay in this posture for 5-10 minutes, concentrating on deepening your breath and building a sensation of serenity and relaxation.

Routine 4: Full Body Flow

This program mixes dynamic movements and static holds to produce a fluid sequence that addresses the entire body and improves general well-being.

1. Seated Sun Salutation:

- • - Begin by sitting tall in your chair with your feet flat on the floor and your hands resting on your thighs.

- • - Inhale to stretch your arms above, bringing your palms together.

- • - Exhale to tilt forward from your hips, bringing your chest towards your thighs and your hands towards the floor.

- • - Inhale to stretch your spine and pull your chest forward, entering into a sitting backbend.

- • - Exhale to circle your spine and lower your chin into your chest, going into a sitting forward fold.

- • - Continue to go through this cycle with your breath, flowing naturally and attentively.

2. Seated Warrior Flow:

- • - Sit tall in your chair with your feet flat on the floor and your spine straight.

- • - Inhale to stretch your arms above, bringing your palms together.

- - Exhale to bend your elbows and cactus your arms, expanding your chest and pulling your shoulder blades together.

- - Inhale to straighten your arms and stretch them aloft, lengthening across the sides of your body.

- - Exhale to rotate to the right, resting your left hand on the outside of your right leg and your right hand on the back of the chair.

- - Inhale to return to center, then exhale to repeat on the other side.

- • - Continue to flow between these two postures with your breath, flowing with ease and fluidity.

3. Seated Chair Flow:

- • - Begin by sitting tall in your chair with your feet flat on the floor and your hands resting on your thighs.

- • - Inhale to stretch your arms above, bringing your palms together.

- • - Exhale to tilt forward from your hips, bringing your chest towards your thighs and your hands towards the floor.

- - Inhale to stretch your spine and pull your chest forward, entering into a sitting backbend.

- - Exhale to circle your spine and lower your chin into your chest, going into a sitting forward fold.

- - Continue to flow between these two postures with your breath, flowing with grace and fluidity.

Routine 5: Balance and Stability

This program focuses on developing balance and stability, enhancing core strength, and generating a sense of groundedness and present.

1. Seated Tree Pose:

- - Begin by sitting tall in your chair with your feet flat on the floor and your spine straight.

- - Shift your weight into your left foot and elevate your right foot off the floor, putting the sole of your right foot against the inside of your left calf or thigh.

- - Press your foot firmly into your leg and your leg back into your foot, establishing a secure and balanced position.

- • - Bring your hands together at your heart center, or stretch them overhead for an extra challenge.

- • - Hold the posture for 3-5 breaths, feeling anchored and grounded through your standing leg.

- • - Exhale to drop your right foot down to the floor and return to a sitting posture, then repeat on the opposite side.

2. Seated Warrior III:

- • - Begin by sitting tall in your chair with your feet flat on the floor and your spine straight.

- • - Shift your weight into your left foot and stretch your right leg straight back behind you, maintaining your toes pointing towards the floor.

- • - Inhale to stretch your arms above, bringing your palms together.

- • - Exhale to hinge forward from your hips, bringing your chest parallel to the floor and your arms beside your ears.

- - Hold the posture for 3-5 breaths, experiencing a sense of strength and stability through your standing leg and core.

- - Inhale to return to a sitting position, then repeat on the opposite side.

3. Seated Eagle Pose:

- - Begin by sitting tall in your chair with your feet flat on the floor and your spine straight.

- - Inhale to stretch your arms out to the sides, parallel to the floor.

- - Exhale to cross your right arm across your left, bending your elbows and bringing the backs of your hands together.

- - If feasible, wrap your right forearm over your left forearm, bringing your hands together.

- - Lift your elbows slightly and press your hands away from your face, experiencing a stretch across the shoulders and upper back.

- •   - Hold the posture for 3-5 breaths, feeling a sense of compression and expansion through the upper body.

- •   - Inhale to release your arms back to your sides, then repeat on the other side.

4. Seated Half Moon Pose:
- • - Begin by sitting erect in your chair with your feet flat on the floor and your spine straight.

- •   - Inhale to reach your right arm up towards the ceiling, stretching through the right half of your body.

- - Exhale to lean softly to the left, bringing your right hand towards the floor and your left hand towards the ceiling.

- - Keep both hips anchored on the chair and both feet flat on the floor.

- - Hold the posture for 3-5 breaths, experiencing a deep stretch across the right side of your body.

- - Inhale to return to center, then exhale to repeat on the other side.

5. Seated Dancer Pose:

- - Begin by sitting tall in your chair with your feet flat on the floor and your spine straight.

- - Inhale to raise your right arm up towards the sky, and bend your right elbow, bringing your right hand towards your upper back.

- - Exhale to extend your left hand back and take hold of your right ankle or foot.

- - Press your foot into your hand and your hand into your foot, experiencing a deep stretch through the front of your body.

- - Hold the posture for 3-5 breaths, feeling a sense of expansion and opening through the chest and shoulders.

- - Inhale to release your foot back to the floor, then exhale to repeat on the opposite side.

Routine 6: Core and Abdominal Strengt

This program focuses on strengthening the core and abdominal muscles, improving posture, and promoting stability and balance.

1. Seated Boat Pose:

- - Begin by sitting tall in your chair with your feet flat on the floor and your Keep the spine straight. Lean back slightly and elevate your feet off the floor, making your shins parallel to the ground.

- - Engage your core and stretch your arms forward, reaching them alongside your legs.

- - Hold the posture for 3-5 breaths, feeling a sensation of activation and engagement through the core and legs.

- - Exhale to lower your feet down to the floor and return to a sitting position.

2. Seated Crunches:

- - Begin by sitting erect in your chair with your feet flat on the floor and your spine straight.

- - Interlace your fingers behind your head and draw your elbows wide.

- - Exhale to engage your core and pull your chest towards your thighs, bringing your elbows towards your knees.

- - Inhale to descend back down to the beginning position.

- - Repeat for 10-15 reps, moving with control and attention.

3. Seated Leg Lifts:

- • - Begin by sitting tall in your chair Position your feet flat on the floor and your spine straight. Put your hands on the sides of your chair for support.

- • - Exhale to engage your core and lift your legs off the floor, bringing your knees towards your chest.

- • - Inhale to drop your legs back down towards the floor, but don't let them contact.

- • - Repeat for 10-15 reps, moving with control and attention.

4. Seated Bicycle Crunches:

- • - Begin by sitting tall in your chair with your feet flat on the floor and your spine straight.

- • - Interlace your fingers behind your head and draw your elbows wide.

- • - Exhale to engage your core and pull your chest towards your thighs, bringing your right elbow towards your left knee while extending your right leg.

- ● - Inhale to return to the beginning position, then exhale to repeat on the opposite side.

- ● - Continue to alternate sides for 10-15 repetitions, moving with control and attention.

5. Seated Twists:

- ● - Begin by sitting tall in your chair with your feet flat on the floor and your spine straight.

- ● - Place your hands on the sides of your chair for support.

- - Exhale to engage your core and rotate to the right, bringing your left elbow towards your right knee.

- - Inhale to return to center, then exhale to twist to the left, bringing your right elbow towards your left knee.

- - Continue to alternate sides for 10-15 repetitions, moving with control and attention.

Routine 7: Relaxation and Restoration

This program focuses on relaxation and restoration, helping to reduce stress, quiet the mind, and enhance general well-being.

1. Seated Relaxation Pose:

* - Sit tall in your chair with your feet flat on the floor and your hands resting on your thighs.

* - Close your eyes and take a few deep breaths, inhaling with your nose and expelling through your mouth.

- • - Allow your body to relax completely, releasing any tension or tightness with each breath.

- • - Stay in this posture for 5-10 minutes, concentrating on deepening your breath and generating a sensation of peace and relaxation.

2. Seated Guided Meditation:
- • - Sit tall in your chair with your feet flat on the floor and your hands resting on your thighs.

- • - Close your eyes and take a few deep breaths to focus yourself.

- - Begin to focus on your breath, experiencing the sensation of each inhale and exhale.

- - As you continue to breathe deeply, envision a location of calm and serenity, such as a serene beach or a quiet forest.

- - Allow yourself to fully engage in this vision, observing the sights, sounds, and sensations of your imagined environment.

- - Stay in this state of relaxation for 5-10 minutes, allowing yourself to let go of whatever stress or tension you may be holding onto.

3. Seated Body Scan:

- - Sit tall in your chair with your feet flat on the floor and your hands resting on your thighs.

- - Close your eyes and take a few deep breaths to focus yourself.

- - Begin to bring your awareness to different regions of your body, starting with your feet and progressing upwards towards your head.

- ●   - Notice any feelings or regions of tension as you scan each portion of your body, but try not to evaluate or analyze them.

- ●   - Simply watch whatever comes with a spirit of wonder and acceptance.

- ●   - Continue to inspect your body from head to toe, taking your time and inhaling deeply.

- ●   - Once you've done the scan, spend a few seconds to remain in silence and examine how your body feels as a whole.

Routine 8: Chair Yoga for Every Body

This program includes tweaks and variations to make chair yoga accessible to practitioners of various ages, abilities, and fitness levels.

1. Seated Mountain Pose:

- - Begin by sitting erect in your chair with your feet flat on the floor and your hands resting on your thighs.

- - Close your eyes and take a few deep breaths, inhaling with your nose and expelling through your mouth.

- - Visualize yourself as a towering, beautiful mountain, planted securely into the soil below.

- - Feel the power and stability of the mountain inside you, stabilizing you and supporting you as you progress through your exercise.

- - Stay in this posture for 5-10 breaths, concentrating on deepening your breath and connecting with your inner power.

2. Seated Cat-Cow Stretch:

- - Begin by sitting tall in your chair with your feet flat on the floor and your hands resting on your thighs.

- - Inhale to arch your back and elevate your chest towards the ceiling (Cow), pulling your shoulder blades together.

- - Exhale to circle your spine and tuck your chin into your chest (Cat), squeezing your hands into your thighs and rounding your upper back.

- ● - Continue to move between these two postures with your breath, moving easily and attentively.

- ● - If you have limited mobility or flexibility in your spine, you may alter this position by just focusing on the flow of your breath and imagining the forms of Cow and Cat in your mind.

3. Seated Warrior II:
- ● - Sit tall in your chair with your feet flat on the floor and your spine straight.

- •   - Extend your right leg out to the side, keeping your knee bent and your foot flat on the floor.

- •   - Turn your body towards the right, bringing your right hand to rest on your right thigh and your left hand to rest on your left thigh.

- •   - Lift your left arm up towards the ceiling, stretching it overhead and then out to the side.

- •   - Gaze towards your left hand, experiencing a sense of power and resolve in your Warrior II position.

- • - Hold the position for 3-5 breaths, then swap sides and repeat on the left.

4. Seated Forward Fold:

- • - Begin by sitting erect in your chair with your feet flat on the floor and your hands resting on your thighs.

- • - Inhale to extend your spine, then exhale to tilt forward from your hips, bringing your chest towards your thighs and your hands towards the floor.

- • - Allow your head to hang heavy and your shoulders to relax.

- • - If you have limited flexibility in your hamstrings or lower back, you may adjust this posture by bending your knees slightly or laying a cushion or folded blanket on your thighs to support your upper body.

5. Seated Twist:

- • - Sit tall in your chair with your feet flat on the floor and your spine straight.

- - Inhale to extend your spine, then exhale to rotate to the right, resting your left hand on the outside of your right leg and your right hand on the back of the chair.

- - Gently press into the chair with your right hand to deepen the twist, and move your eyes over your right shoulder.

- - If you have restricted mobility in your spine or shoulders, you may adjust this posture by simply moving your body towards the right and resting your hands on your thighs for support.

This complete chair yoga program covers a varied range of postures to help your weight reduction quest. Each exercise has distinct advantages for the body and mind, helping you grow strength, flexibility, balance, and relaxation. By implementing these techniques into your daily routine, you may boost your general well-being and reach your weight reduction objectives with ease and fun.

CHAPTER 6

NUTRITION AND DIET TIPS FOR EFFECTIVE WEIGHT LOSS WITH CHAIR YOGA

In this part, we will address the relevance of nutrition and food in conjunction with chair yoga for optimal weight loss. We will look into the significance of adequate nutrition in supporting your body's needs, supplying energy for physical activity, and boosting general health and well-being. Additionally, we will examine essential nutritional concepts and practical suggestions for implementing good eating habits into your daily.

Understanding Nutrition: To begin our journey into nutrition and weight reduction, it's vital to grasp the basic concepts of nutrition. We will investigate the three macronutrients — carbs, proteins, and fats – and their roles in the body. We'll also cover the importance of micronutrients, such as vitamins and minerals, for general health and vigor. Understanding the foundations of nutrition can enable you to make educated dietary choices that support your weight reduction objectives.

Balanced Diet: A balanced diet is vital for obtaining and maintaining a healthy weight. In this part, we will explain the components of a balanced diet, including whole grains, lean meats, healthy fats, fruits, and vegetables. We'll explore portion management and mindful eating methods to help you manage your calorie intake successfully. By adopting a balanced diet, you may fuel your body with the nutrition it needs while boosting weight reduction and general wellness.

Hydration: Proper hydration is essential for overall health and well-being, especially during weight loss. In this section, we will explore the importance of staying hydrated and its impact on metabolism, digestion, and energy levels. We'll discuss how to calculate your daily fluid needs and practical tips for staying hydrated throughout the day. By prioritizing hydration, you can support your weight loss efforts and optimize your overall health.

Meal Planning: Meal planning is a valuable tool for achieving your weight loss goals and maintaining a healthy lifestyle. In this section, we will discuss the benefits of meal planning and provide practical tips for getting started. We'll explore strategies for batch cooking, prepping ingredients in advance, and creating balanced meals that support your nutritional needs. With proper meal planning, you can save time, reduce stress, and make healthier food choices.

Mindful Eating: Mindful eating is a powerful practice that can enhance your relationship with food and support your weight loss journey. In this section, we will explore the concept of mindful eating and its benefits for weight management.

We'll discuss techniques for practicing mindful eating, such as paying attention to hunger and fullness cues, savoring each bite, and avoiding distractions while eating. By cultivating mindfulness around food, you can make more conscious choices and develop a healthier relationship with eating.

Nutrition and Exercise: Nutrition and exercise go hand in hand when it comes to achieving weight loss goals. In this section, we will explore the relationship between nutrition and exercise and how they complement each other. We'll discuss the importance of fueling your body properly before and after exercise, as well as strategies for optimizing your nutrition to support physical activity. By aligning your nutrition and exercise habits, you can maximize your weight loss results and improve your overall fitness level.

Healthy Snacking: Snacking can be a valuable part of a healthy diet when done mindfully. In this section, we will explore the importance of healthy snacking for weight loss and provide practical tips for choosing nutritious snacks. We'll discuss healthy snack options that are rich in protein, fiber, and healthy fats to keep you feeling satisfied and energized between meals. By incorporating healthy snacks into your diet, you can curb cravings, prevent overeating, and support your weight loss efforts.

nutrition plays a critical role in achieving and maintaining weight loss, especially when combined with chair yoga. By understanding the fundamentals of nutrition, adopting a balanced diet, staying hydrated, meal planning, practicing mindful eating, and aligning your nutrition with exercise, you can optimize your weight loss results and improve your overall health and well-being. With these nutrition and diet tips, you can embark on a journey towards a healthier, happier you.

CHAPTER 7

OVERCOMING CHALLENGES AND PLATEAUS IN YOUR WEIGHT LOSS JOURNEY WITH CHAIR YOGA

on a weight loss journey with chair yoga can be both empowering and rewarding. However, along the way, you may encounter challenges and plateaus that can hinder your progress. In this section, we will explore common obstacles faced during weight loss and how to overcome them with resilience and determination.

We'll discuss strategies for navigating challenges and breaking through plateaus to achieve your goals and maintain long-term success.

Understanding Challenges and Plateaus:

Before diving into strategies for overcoming challenges and plateaus, it's essential to understand what they are and why they occur. Challenges can arise from various factors, including lifestyle habits, emotional triggers, environmental influences, and physiological responses. Plateaus occur when your body reaches a state of equilibrium and stops responding to your weight loss efforts, leading to a temporary halt in progress. By understanding the root causes of challenges and plateaus, you can develop targeted strategies for overcoming them effectively.

Mindset and Motivation: Maintaining a positive mindset and staying motivated are crucial for overcoming challenges and plateaus in your weight loss journey. In this section, we will explore the power of mindset and motivation and how they influence your ability to overcome obstacles. We'll discuss techniques for cultivating a resilient mindset, setting realistic goals, and staying focused on your vision for success. By harnessing the power of your mind, you can overcome any challenge that comes your way and stay motivated to achieve your weight loss goals.

Adaptability and Flexibility: Flexibility and adaptability are essential qualities for navigating challenges and plateaus in your weight loss journey. In this section, we will discuss the importance of being flexible in your approach to weight loss and adapting to changing circumstances. We'll explore strategies for adjusting your workout routine, modifying your diet plan, and trying new techniques to break through plateaus and overcome obstacles. By remaining open-minded and willing to adapt, you can find creative solutions to overcome any challenge that arises.

Problem-Solving Skills: Developing problem-solving skills is essential for overcoming challenges and plateaus in your weight loss journey. In this section, we will explore effective problem-solving techniques and how to apply them to common obstacles. We'll discuss strategies for identifying barriers to weight loss, brainstorming potential solutions, and implementing action plans to address challenges head-on. By honing your problem-solving skills, you can approach obstacles with confidence and find practical solutions to overcome them.

Support System: Having a strong support system can make a significant difference in your ability to overcome challenges and plateaus in your weight loss journey. In this section, we will discuss the importance of seeking support from friends, family, and peers who understand your goals and can offer encouragement and guidance. We'll explore how to build a support network that empowers you to stay motivated, accountable, and resilient in the face of obstacles. By surrounding yourself with positive influences, you can overcome challenges and plateaus with greater ease and confidence.

Self-Care Practices: Practicing self-care is essential for maintaining physical, mental, and emotional well-being during your weight loss journey. In this section, we will explore self-care practices that can help you overcome challenges and plateaus with grace and resilience. We'll discuss techniques for managing stress, prioritizing rest and relaxation, and nurturing your body and mind. By incorporating self-care into your daily routine, you can replenish your energy, boost your mood, and cultivate resilience to overcome any obstacle that comes your way.

Continuous Learning and Growth: Embracing a mindset of continuous learning and growth is essential for overcoming challenges and plateaus in your weight loss journey. In this section, we will discuss the importance of seeking knowledge, experimenting with new approaches, and embracing failure as an opportunity for growth. We'll explore how to stay curious, open-minded, and resilient in the face of setbacks, knowing that every challenge is an opportunity to learn and evolve. By embracing a growth mindset, you can overcome obstacles with confidence and continue to progress towards your weight loss goals.

overcoming challenges and plateaus in your weight loss journey with chair yoga requires resilience, determination, and a positive mindset. By understanding the root causes of challenges and plateaus, cultivating a resilient mindset, staying adaptable and flexible, honing problem-solving skills, seeking support, practicing self-care, and embracing continuous learning and growth, you can overcome any obstacle that comes your way and achieve long-term success in your weight loss journey. With perseverance and dedication, you can overcome challenges and plateaus with grace and resilience, reaching your goals and living your best life.

CHAPTER 8

Incorporating chair yoga into your daily life can have profound benefits for your physical, mental, and emotional well-being. By integrating simple chair yoga practices into your routine, you can reduce stress, improve flexibility and strength, enhance mindfulness, and cultivate a greater sense of overall vitality. In this section, we will explore practical strategies for incorporating chair yoga into various aspects of your daily life, from your morning routine to your workday and bedtime rituals.

Morning Routine: Starting your day with a gentle chair yoga practice can set a positive tone for the rest of the day. Begin by sitting comfortably in your chair with your feet flat on the floor and your spine straight. Take a few deep breaths to center yourself and awaken your body and mind. Then, engage in a series of gentle stretches and movements to release tension and increase circulation. You can incorporate movements such as neck rolls, shoulder shrugs, side stretches, and spinal twists to awaken your muscles and joints and prepare your body for the day ahead.

Midday Breaks: Taking short breaks throughout the day to practice chair yoga can help alleviate stress, boost energy levels, and enhance focus and productivity. Schedule brief chair yoga sessions during your breaks at work or while studying at home. Focus on gentle stretches and breathing exercises to relax your body and calm your mind. You can practice seated forward folds, chest openers, and deep breathing exercises to release tension and recenter yourself amidst the demands of the day. These mini yoga breaks can help you maintain a sense of balance and well-being throughout the day.

Workstation Yoga: Incorporating chair yoga into your workstation setup can help alleviate the physical strain associated with prolonged sitting and computer use. Set up your workstation ergonomically, with your chair positioned at the appropriate height and distance from your desk. Throughout the day, take short breaks to practice chair yoga poses and stretches to release tension in your neck, shoulders, back, and wrists. You can incorporate movements such as wrist circles, seated cat-cow stretches, and shoulder rolls to counteract the effects of sitting and typing for extended periods.

Mindful Eating: Practicing chair yoga can also enhance your experience of mealtimes by promoting mindfulness and conscious eating. Before meals, take a moment to center yourself and connect with your breath. As you eat, focus on savoring each bite and paying attention to the flavors, textures, and sensations of the food. You can practice mindful breathing exercises between bites to slow down your pace of eating and tune into your body's hunger and fullness cues. By incorporating mindfulness into your eating habits, you can cultivate a greater sense of satisfaction and enjoyment from your meals.

Evening Relaxation: Ending your day with a gentle chair yoga practice can help you unwind, release tension, and prepare your body and mind for restful sleep. Before bedtime, find a quiet space where you can sit comfortably in your chair without distractions. Engage in a series of relaxing stretches and breathing exercises to soothe your nervous system and promote relaxation. Focus on movements that target areas of tension, such as gentle neck stretches, shoulder releases, and spinal twists. You can also practice deep breathing exercises and progressive muscle relaxation to calm your mind and body before bedtime.

Incorporating chair yoga into your daily life doesn't have to be complicated or time-consuming. By integrating simple chair yoga practices into your morning routine, midday breaks, workstation setup, mealtimes, and evening relaxation rituals, you can experience the profound benefits of yoga in your everyday life. Whether you're looking to reduce stress, improve flexibility, enhance mindfulness, or simply add more movement into your day, chair yoga offers accessible and effective tools for promoting health and well-being. So why not give it a try and see how chair yoga can enhance your daily life?

CHAPTER 9

ADVANCED CHAIR YOGA TECHNIQUES

Alignment and Body Awareness: In advanced chair yoga, practitioners deepen their understanding of alignment principles and body awareness to refine their practice and prevent injury. Focus on aligning the body's various parts in optimal positions to facilitate ease and efficiency of movement. Pay attention to the subtle cues and sensations in the body, cultivating a heightened awareness of how each movement affects different muscle groups and joints. Through mindful alignment and body awareness, practitioners can enhance their practice and experience greater freedom and ease in movement.

Breath Control and Pranayama: Advanced chair yoga incorporates advanced breath control techniques, known as pranayama, to deepen the connection between the body and mind and enhance the flow of vital energy throughout the body. Explore various pranayama techniques, such as ujjayi breath, kapalabhati, and nadi shodhana, to regulate the breath, calm the mind, and invigorate the body. Practice synchronized breathing with movement to create a seamless flow of energy and cultivate a sense of presence and focus in your practice.

Seated Meditation and Mindfulness: Advanced chair yoga includes seated meditation and mindfulness practices to cultivate inner peace, clarity, and insight. Set aside dedicated time for seated meditation, focusing on cultivating a calm and focused mind amidst the distractions of everyday life. Explore different meditation techniques, such as breath awareness, loving-kindness meditation, and body scan meditation, to develop greater self-awareness and emotional resilience. Cultivate mindfulness in your daily activities, bringing awareness to the present moment with openness, curiosity, and acceptance.

Advanced Asana Variations: In advanced chair yoga, practitioners explore advanced variations of traditional yoga poses to deepen their practice and challenge their strength, flexibility, and balance. Experiment with variations of familiar poses, such as seated forward bends, twists, backbends, and inversions, using the support of the chair to deepen your stretches and refine your alignment. Explore creative sequencing and transitions between poses to cultivate fluidity and grace in your practice. With dedication and patience, advanced practitioners can unlock new levels of mastery and embodiment in their practice.

Yoga Philosophy and Spiritual Inquiry: Advanced chair yoga delves into the rich philosophical and spiritual teachings of yoga to deepen practitioners' understanding of themselves and the world around them. Study classical yoga texts, such as the Yoga Sutras of Patanjali, the

Bhagavad Gita, and the Hatha Yoga Pradipika, to explore profound insights into the nature of the mind, body, and spirit. Reflect on the ethical principles of yoga, such as ahimsa (non-violence), satya (truthfulness), and santosha (contentment), and contemplate how these teachings can be applied in your daily life.

Advanced Relaxation and Yoga Nidra: Advanced chair yoga includes advanced relaxation techniques and yoga nidra (yogic sleep) practices to promote deep relaxation, healing, and rejuvenation. Explore progressive relaxation techniques to release tension and promote physical and mental relaxation systematically. Practice yoga nidra to enter a state of conscious deep sleep, where you can access deeper layers of the subconscious mind and experience profound states of relaxation, insight, and transformation. Incorporate visualization, affirmation, and sankalpa (intention-setting) into your relaxation practice to harness the power of the mind for healing and manifestation.

Advanced Pranayama and Meditation: In advanced chair yoga, practitioners deepen their pranayama and meditation practices to access higher states of consciousness and spiritual awakening.

Experiment with advanced pranayama techniques, such as bhastrika (bellows breath), surya bheda (right nostril breathing), and chandra bheda (left nostril breathing), to balance and harmonize the flow of prana (life force energy) in the body. Dive deeper into meditation, exploring advanced meditation techniques, such as transcendental meditation, kundalini meditation, and vipassana meditation, to cultivate inner stillness, clarity, and insight. Through advanced pranayama and meditation practices, practitioners can awaken to their true nature and experience a profound sense of unity and interconnectedness with all of life.

Advanced chair yoga techniques offer practitioners an opportunity to deepen their practice and explore new dimensions of physical, mental, and spiritual well-being. By integrating alignment and body awareness, breath control and pranayama, seated meditation and mindfulness, advanced asana variations, yoga philosophy and spiritual inquiry, advanced relaxation and yoga nidra, and advanced pranayama and meditation practices into their practice, practitioners can unlock new levels of mastery, insight, and transformation on their yoga journey. So why not embark on the journey of advanced chair yoga and discover the limitless potential of your body, mind, and spirit?

CHAPTER 10

CHAIR YOGA FOR LONG-TERM WEIGHT

Management: Sustainable Practices for Health and Wellness In today's fast-paced world, maintaining a healthy weight can be a challenge for many individuals. However, with the practice of chair yoga, long-term weight management becomes not only achievable but sustainable. Chair yoga offers accessible and effective tools for improving physical fitness, reducing stress, and promoting mindfulness, all of which are essential components of a successful weight management plan. In this comprehensive guide, we will explore the principles of chair yoga for long-term weight management and provide practical strategies for incorporating chair yoga into your daily routine to support your health and wellness goals.

Understanding Long-Term Weight Management: Long-term weight management is about more than just shedding pounds; it's about adopting sustainable lifestyle habits that support overall health and well-being. Successful weight management involves a combination of regular physical activity, mindful eating, stress management, and self-care practices. Chair yoga offers a holistic approach to weight management by addressing these key areas of health and wellness, making it an ideal complement to traditional weight loss strategies.

Benefits of Chair Yoga for Weight Management: Chair yoga offers numerous benefits for weight management, including improved flexibility, strength, balance, and cardiovascular health. By practicing chair yoga regularly, individuals can increase their physical fitness levels, burn calories, and build lean muscle mass, all of which contribute to a healthy weight. Additionally, chair yoga promotes relaxation and stress reduction, helping individuals manage emotional eating and cravings more effectively. The mindfulness practices incorporated into chair yoga also support mindful eating habits, encouraging individuals to eat more intuitively and make healthier food choices.

Incorporating Chair Yoga into Your Daily Routine: Incorporating chair yoga into your daily routine is simple and convenient, making it accessible to individuals of all ages and fitness levels. Begin by setting aside dedicated time each day for chair yoga practice, starting with just a few minutes and gradually increasing the duration as you become more comfortable. You can practice chair yoga at home, in the office, or even while traveling, making it easy to stay consistent with your practice regardless of your schedule. With regular practice, you'll soon start to notice the physical, mental, and emotional benefits of chair yoga for weight management.

.

Chair Yoga Poses for Weight Management: Chair yoga poses are gentle yet effective movements that can help individuals build strength, improve flexibility, and increase energy levels. Some beneficial chair yoga poses for weight management include seated forward bends, spinal twists, side stretches, and gentle backbends. These poses target key muscle groups, such as the core, back, shoulders, and legs, helping individuals tone and sculpt their bodies while burning calories. Additionally, chair yoga poses can help improve posture and alignment, reducing the risk of injury and promoting overall physical health.

Mindful Eating Practices: In addition to physical movement, chair yoga emphasizes the importance of mindful eating practices for weight management. Mindful eating involves paying attention to hunger and mindfulness, or just bring more movement into your day, chair yoga offers accessible and effective techniques for enhancing health and well-being. So why not give it a try and discover how chair yoga may boost your daily life?

Stress Management and Emotional Well-Being: Stress management is a vital component of long-term weight control, since persistent stress can contribute to emotional eating, cravings, and weight gain. Chair yoga offers excellent stress management strategies, such as deep breathing exercises, relaxation positions, and meditation, that assist individuals lower stress levels and increase emotional well-being. By implementing these techniques into their daily routine, individuals may create a better feeling of tranquility, resilience, and inner peace, making it easier to cope with the challenges of everyday life without resorting to food for consolation.

Building a Support Network: Building a support network is vital for long-term weight control success, as having a strong support system may give encouragement, accountability, and inspiration. Chair yoga courses offer a supportive community setting where individuals may interact with like-minded folks who share similar health and fitness goals. Additionally, internet tools, such as forums, social media groups, and virtual yoga communities, give chances for individuals to interact with others, exchange experiences, and seek support on their weight control journey. By surrounding oneself with good influences, individuals may stay motivated and devoted to their health and fitness goals.

Chair yoga offers a holistic approach to long-term weight control, addressing physical, mental, and emotional aspects of health and wellness. By including chair yoga into your daily routine, you may increase flexibility, strength, and balance, reduce stress, and develop mindful eating habits, all of which contribute to sustainable weight management. Whether you're wanting to lose weight, maintain a healthy weight, or simply enhance your general well-being, chair yoga offers accessible and effective methods for accomplishing your health and wellness objectives. So why not go on the path of chair yoga for long-term weight control and explore the transformational potential of this gentle yet powerful practice?

Seated yoga gives a holistic approach to long-term weight control, addressing physical, mental, and emotional aspects of health and fitness. By including chair yoga into your daily routine, you may increase flexibility, strength, and balance, reduce stress, and develop mindful eating habits, all of which contribute to sustainable weight management. Whether you're wanting to lose weight, maintain a healthy weight, or simply enhance your general well-being, chair yoga offers accessible and effective methods for accomplishing your health and wellness objectives. So why not go on the path of chair yoga for long-term weight control and explore the transformational potential of this gentle yet powerful practice

CONCLUSION,

chair yoga emerges as a valuable technique for achieving long-term weight control and general well-being. Through its accessible and compassionate approach, chair yoga allows individuals of all ages and fitness levels the chance to enhance their physical, mental, and emotional health in sustainable ways.

One of the important takeaways from investigating chair yoga for weight loss is its versatility and adaptability. Chair yoga may be performed anywhere, anytime, making it accessible to anyone with hectic schedules, limited mobility, or physical disabilities. Whether at home, at the workplace, or even while traveling, chair yoga offers a handy method to incorporate movement, mindfulness, and relaxation into daily life.

Furthermore, chair yoga stresses the significance of holistic health, addressing not only the physical elements of weight control but also the mental and emotional components. By combining mindful eating habits, stress management strategies, and self-care activities into their daily routine, individuals may build a more balanced and sustainable approach to weight control.

Moreover, chair yoga develops a feeling of community and support, giving individuals with a welcoming setting where they may interact with others, exchange experiences, and seek encouragement on their weight control path. Whether in a group class or online community, the friendship and encouragement found in chair yoga environments may give important support and inspiration.

Additionally, chair yoga provides folks a sense of control and autonomy over their health and well-being. By practicing chair yoga frequently, individuals may develop increased self-awareness, resilience, and self-efficacy, enabling them to make better choices and handle problems with confidence and grace.

Overall, chair yoga stands out as a gentle yet strong exercise for long-term weight control. Its accessibility, adaptability, and comprehensive approach make it a great supplement to standard weight reduction treatments, allowing patients a sustainable route to increased health and wellness. By adopting chair yoga into their daily routine and embracing its transforming potential, individuals may begin on a path of self-discovery, empowerment, and sustainable change. So why not take the first step towards a healthier, happier you with chair yoga for long-term weight management?